Emphysema Explained

Your Complete Guide to Understanding and Managing Emphysema

Isabella White

Disclaimer: *The information contained in this book is based on the research, opinions, and experiences of the author. It is not intended to replace professional medical advice or treatment. The reader should regularly consult a physician for any health issues and always seek the advice of a physician before modifying diet, supplement, or exercise regimens.*

The author and publisher shall have neither liability nor responsibility to any person or entity concerning any loss or damage related to the information contained in this book. The information provided is general in nature and may not apply to every individual. Any reliance on the information contained herein is solely at the reader's risk.

Contents

Chapter 5

Support and Resources ______ **84**

Conclusion ______ **104**

Overview

Emphysema is a long-term respiratory condition that affects millions of people globally. It is a progressive disease that leads to breathing difficulties as a result of damage to the tiny air sacs (alveoli) in the lungs. This damage ultimately reduces the overall lung capacity and causes shortness of breath.

If you or a loved one has been diagnosed with emphysema, this book will provide you with a comprehensive guide to understanding this condition and actively managing symptoms and lifestyle factors. While emphysema is a serious disease, many people can live full and fulfilling lives with proper treatment and a positive mindset.

In the following chapters, we will explore the causes and types of emphysema, go over conventional medical treatments, discuss lifestyle changes and alternative therapies, provide tips on building a support system, and outline ways to set goals and live your best life. You will gain a deeper understanding of what happens to the lungs in emphysema and get actionable advice on improving your breathing, everyday functioning, diet, exercise routine, and emotional health.

It's normal to feel shocked, worried, or overwhelmed after an emphysema diagnosis. This book will empower you with knowledge and serve as a helpful resource as you navigate life with this condition. With the proper education, support system, and proactive approach, it is possible to manage emphysema symptoms successfully. This guide aims to help you on that path.

Chapter 1

Introduction to Emphysema

What is Emphysema?

Emphysema is a lung disease that is chronic and progressive in nature. It primarily affects the air sacs, also known as alveoli, in the lungs. Emphysema is classified as a type of chronic obstructive pulmonary disease (COPD). The disease is characterized by the destruction of the walls of the alveoli, which leads to the formation of larger, less efficient air spaces. This results in a decrease in the surface area that is available for oxygen and carbon dioxide exchange, which further leads to difficulty in breathing.

The main cause of emphysema is long-term exposure to irritants, such as cigarette smoke, air pollution, chemical fumes, and dust. In rare cases, a genetic condition called alpha-1 antitrypsin deficiency can predispose individuals to developing emphysema at a younger age.

The destruction of the alveoli in emphysema is primarily caused by an imbalance between protease enzymes and antiprotease enzymes in the lungs. Protease enzymes, such as elastase, break down the connective tissue in the lungs, while antiprotease enzymes, such as alpha-1 antitrypsin, help to protect the lungs from this damage. In individuals with emphysema, there is an excess of protease enzymes or a deficiency of antiprotease enzymes, leading to the destruction of the alveolar walls.

As the disease progresses, the lungs lose their elasticity, making it difficult for them to expand and contract properly during breathing. This results in a decrease in the amount of oxygen that can enter the bloodstream and a buildup of carbon dioxide, leading to symptoms such as shortness of breath, wheezing, coughing, and fatigue.

Emphysema is a chronic condition, meaning that it cannot be cured. However, with proper management and treatment, the progression of the disease can be slowed down, and symptoms can be alleviated. Individuals with emphysema need to work closely with their healthcare team to develop a personalized treatment plan.

In addition to cigarette smoke and other irritants, several risk factors can increase the likelihood of developing emphysema. These include a history of smoking, exposure to secondhand smoke, occupational exposure to certain chemicals or dust, a family history of emphysema, and a history of respiratory infections.

It is estimated that approximately 3.5 million people in the United States have been diagnosed with emphysema, and it is more common in individuals over the age of 40. Men are also more likely to develop emphysema than women, although the gap is narrowing due to increased smoking rates among women.

Causes and Risk Factors

Emphysema is a chronic lung condition that is primarily caused by long-term exposure to irritants that damage the air sacs in the lungs. The main cause of emphysema is cigarette smoking, which is responsible for about 80–90% of all cases. However, other factors can contribute to the development of emphysema as well.

Cigarette Smoking

Cigarette smoke contains thousands of harmful chemicals, including nicotine, tar, and carbon monoxide. When these chemicals are inhaled, they can cause inflammation and damage to the delicate air sacs in the lungs. Over time, this damage leads to the destruction of the air sacs and the development of emphysema.

It's important to note that not all smokers develop emphysema, but the risk is significantly higher for those who smoke. The longer and more heavily a person smokes, the greater their risk of developing emphysema. Quitting smoking is the most effective way to prevent further damage to the lungs and slow the progression of the disease.

Environmental Factors

In addition to cigarette smoke, exposure to other environmental irritants can also contribute to the development of emphysema. These irritants include:

- **Secondhand smoke:** Breathing in the smoke from other people's cigarettes can be just as harmful as smoking itself. Secondhand smoke contains many of the same harmful chemicals as firsthand smoke and can cause lung damage over time.
- **Air pollution:** Living in areas with high levels of air pollution, such as cities with heavy traffic or industrial areas, can increase the risk of developing emphysema. The pollutants in the air can irritate the lungs and lead to inflammation and damage.
- **Occupational exposure:** Certain occupations, such as coal mining, construction work, and

manufacturing, expose workers to harmful substances like dust, chemicals, and fumes. Prolonged exposure to these substances can increase the risk of developing emphysema.

Genetic Factors

While smoking and environmental factors are the primary causes of emphysema, there is also a genetic component to the disease. Some individuals are born with a deficiency of a protein called alpha-1 antitrypsin (AAT), which helps protect the lungs from damage. Without enough AAT, the lungs are more susceptible to the harmful effects of irritants like cigarette smoke.

Alpha-1 antitrypsin deficiency (AATD) is a rare genetic condition that affects about 1 in 2,500 individuals. People with AATD are at a significantly higher risk of developing emphysema, even if they have never smoked or been exposed to other environmental irritants. Genetic testing can determine if a person has AATD and can help guide treatment decisions.

Age and Gender

Age and gender can also play a role in the development of emphysema. The risk of developing the disease increases with age, as the lungs naturally lose their elasticity and become more vulnerable to damage. Men are also more likely to develop emphysema than women, although the gap is narrowing as more women take up smoking.

Other Risk Factors

In addition to the main causes and risk factors mentioned above, several other factors can increase the likelihood of developing emphysema. These include:

- **Family history:** Having a family history of emphysema or other lung diseases can increase the risk of developing the condition.
- **Respiratory infections:** Repeated respiratory infections, such as pneumonia or bronchitis, can cause damage to the lungs and increase the risk of emphysema.
- **Asthma:** People with asthma have a higher risk of developing emphysema, especially if their asthma is poorly controlled or they smoke.
- **Chronic bronchitis:** Chronic bronchitis is often associated with emphysema, and the two conditions frequently coexist.
- **HIV infection:** HIV infection can increase the risk of developing emphysema, although the exact reasons for this are not fully understood.

It's important to note that while these factors can increase the risk of developing emphysema, they do not guarantee that a person will develop the disease. Many individuals with one or more risk factors never develop emphysema, while others without any known risk factors may still develop the condition.

Understanding the causes and risk factors can help individuals make informed decisions about their lifestyle choices and take steps to reduce their risk of developing emphysema.

Symptoms and Diagnosis

Emphysema is a chronic lung condition that primarily affects the air sacs in the lungs, known as alveoli. As the disease progresses, these air sacs become damaged and lose their elasticity, making it difficult for the lungs to effectively exchange oxygen and carbon dioxide. This leads to a range of symptoms that can significantly impact a person's quality of life.

Symptoms of Emphysema

The symptoms of emphysema can vary from person to person, depending on the severity of the disease. In the early stages, individuals may not experience any noticeable symptoms. However, as the condition progresses, the following symptoms may become more prominent:

1. **Shortness of breath:** This is one of the most common symptoms of emphysema. It may initially occur during physical exertion but can eventually occur even during rest. As the disease worsens, individuals may find it increasingly difficult to catch their breath.

2. **Chronic cough:** A persistent cough is another common symptom of emphysema. The cough may produce mucus or phlegm and can be worse in the morning or after physical activity.

3. **Wheezing:** Emphysema can cause the airways to narrow, leading to wheezing. Wheezing is a high-pitched whistling sound that occurs when air flows through narrowed airways.

4. **Chest tightness:** Some individuals with emphysema may experience a sensation of tightness or pressure in the chest. This can make breathing even more challenging.

5. **Fatigue:** Due to the decreased efficiency of the lungs, individuals with emphysema often experience fatigue and a lack of energy. This can

make it difficult to perform daily activities and may lead to a decreased quality of life.

6. **Weight loss:** In advanced stages of emphysema, individuals may experience unintentional weight loss. This can be due to the increased energy expenditure required for breathing and the decreased appetite that can accompany the disease.

7. **Recurrent respiratory infections:** Emphysema weakens the immune system's ability to fight off infections, making individuals more susceptible to respiratory infections such as pneumonia and bronchitis.

Diagnosis of Emphysema

Diagnosing emphysema involves a combination of medical history, physical examination, and diagnostic tests. If you are experiencing symptoms that may be indicative of emphysema, it is important to consult a healthcare professional for an accurate diagnosis. The following are some common diagnostic methods used to confirm the presence of emphysema:

1. **Medical history and physical examination:** Your healthcare provider will ask about your symptoms, medical history, and any risk factors you may have

for developing emphysema. They will also listen to your lungs with a stethoscope to check for abnormal breath sounds such as wheezing or crackling.

2. **Pulmonary function tests (PFTs):** PFTs are a series of breathing tests that measure how well your lungs are functioning. The most common test used to diagnose emphysema is spirometry. This test measures the amount of air you can exhale forcefully and how quickly you can do it. It can help determine the severity of airflow obstruction and assess lung function.

3. **Chest X-ray:** A chest X-ray can help identify any abnormalities in the lungs, such as hyperinflation or bullae (large air spaces). While a chest X-ray alone cannot definitively diagnose emphysema, it can provide valuable information to support the diagnosis.

4. **Computed tomography (CT) scan:** A CT scan provides detailed images of the lungs and can help identify emphysema and its extent. It can also help differentiate emphysema from other lung conditions.

5. **Arterial blood gas (ABG) test:** This test measures the levels of oxygen and carbon dioxide in your

blood. It can help assess the severity of respiratory impairment and determine if supplemental oxygen therapy is necessary.

6. **Alpha-1 antitrypsin deficiency testing:** Alpha-1 antitrypsin deficiency is a genetic condition that increases the risk of developing emphysema at an early age. If your healthcare provider suspects this deficiency, they may recommend a blood test to check for it.

It is important to note that emphysema is often diagnosed in conjunction with chronic bronchitis, another form of chronic obstructive pulmonary disease (COPD). The symptoms and diagnostic methods for both conditions are similar, and they often coexist in individuals.

Early diagnosis and intervention are crucial to managing emphysema effectively. If you are experiencing symptoms or have any concerns about your lung health, it is essential to seek medical attention for a proper evaluation and diagnosis.

Treatment Options

When it comes to managing emphysema, there are several treatment options available. The goal of treatment is to relieve symptoms, slow down the progression of the disease, and improve the overall quality of life for individuals with emphysema. Treatment plans are often personalized based on the severity of the condition and the individual's specific needs. In this section, we will explore the various treatment options for emphysema.

1. Medications

Medications play a crucial role in managing emphysema symptoms and preventing complications. The most commonly prescribed medications for emphysema include:

- **Bronchodilators:** These medications help relax the muscles around the airways, making it easier to breathe. They can be inhaled through an inhaler or taken orally. Short-acting bronchodilators provide quick relief during flare-ups, while long-acting bronchodilators are used for daily maintenance.
- **Inhaled Corticosteroids:** These medications help reduce inflammation in the airways, which can help improve breathing. They are often used in combination with bronchodilators for better symptom control.
- **Antibiotics:** In some cases, emphysema can lead to respiratory infections. Antibiotics may be

prescribed to treat these infections and prevent further complications.

- **Vaccinations:** Individuals with emphysema are at a higher risk of developing respiratory infections. Vaccinations, such as the flu vaccine and pneumonia vaccine, are recommended to reduce the risk of these infections.

2. Pulmonary Rehabilitation

Pulmonary rehabilitation is a comprehensive program that combines exercise, education, and support to help individuals with emphysema improve their lung function and overall well-being. The program is usually conducted by a team of healthcare professionals, including respiratory therapists, physical therapists, and dietitians.

The exercise component of pulmonary rehabilitation focuses on improving cardiovascular fitness and strengthening the respiratory muscles. This can help individuals with emphysema become more physically active and reduce breathlessness during daily activities. The education component provides individuals with information about their condition, breathing techniques, and strategies for managing symptoms. Support groups and counseling sessions are also often included to address the emotional and psychological aspects of living with emphysema.

3. Oxygen Therapy

In advanced stages of emphysema, the lungs may not be able to provide enough oxygen to the body. Oxygen therapy involves the use of supplemental oxygen to increase the oxygen levels in the blood. This can help relieve breathlessness, improve exercise tolerance, and enhance overall quality of life.

Oxygen therapy can be administered through various devices, such as nasal cannulas, oxygen masks, or portable oxygen concentrators. The amount of oxygen prescribed will depend on the individual's specific needs, as determined by their healthcare provider.

4. Surgical Options

In some cases, surgical interventions may be considered for individuals with severe emphysema who have not responded well to other treatment options. The two main surgical procedures for emphysema are:

- **Lung Volume Reduction Surgery (LVRS):** This procedure involves removing damaged portions of the lung to improve lung function and reduce breathlessness. It can help improve exercise capacity and quality of life for selected individuals with emphysema.

- **Lung Transplantation:** In severe cases of emphysema, where lung function is severely compromised, a lung transplant may be considered. This involves replacing the diseased lungs with healthy donor lungs. Lung transplantation is a complex procedure and is typically reserved for individuals who meet specific criteria.

5. Managing Exacerbations

Emphysema exacerbations, also known as flare-ups, are episodes of worsening symptoms that can be triggered by respiratory infections or other factors. Managing exacerbations is an important part of emphysema treatment. Treatment during exacerbations may include:

- **Antibiotics:** If the exacerbation is caused by a bacterial infection, antibiotics may be prescribed to treat the infection.

- **Corticosteroids:** Oral or intravenous corticosteroids may be used to reduce inflammation in the airways and improve symptoms.

- **Bronchodilators:** Short-acting bronchodilators may be used to provide immediate relief and improve breathing during exacerbations.
- **Oxygen Therapy:** Supplemental oxygen may be needed during exacerbations to ensure adequate oxygen levels in the blood.

Individuals with emphysema need to work closely with their healthcare team to develop a personalized treatment plan. Regular follow-up appointments and monitoring of symptoms are essential to ensure that the treatment plan is effective and adjusted as needed. With the right treatment approach, individuals with emphysema can effectively manage their condition and lead fulfilling lives.

Chapter 2

Understanding Emphysema

Anatomy of the Lungs

To understand emphysema, it is important to have a basic understanding of the anatomy of the lungs. The lungs are a vital organ responsible for the exchange of oxygen and carbon dioxide in the body. They are located in the chest cavity and are protected by the rib cage.

The lungs are divided into lobes, with the right lung having three lobes and the left lung having two lobes. Each lobe is further divided into smaller sections called lobules. The lobules contain tiny air sacs called alveoli, which are the primary site of gas exchange.

The lungs are surrounded by a thin membrane called the pleura, which helps to protect and lubricate the lungs during breathing. The pleura consists of two layers, the visceral pleura, which covers the surface of the lungs, and the parietal pleura, which lines the chest cavity.

The airways that lead to the lungs begin with the trachea, also known as the windpipe. The trachea branches into two main bronchi, one leading to each lung. Inside the lungs, the bronchi continue to divide into smaller and smaller tubes called bronchioles. The bronchioles eventually end in clusters of alveoli, where the exchange of oxygen and carbon dioxide takes place.

The alveoli are small air sacs in the lungs that are surrounded by a network of tiny blood vessels called capillaries. When we inhale, oxygen from the air diffuses across the thin walls of the alveoli and into the capillaries, where it binds to red blood cells. At the same time, carbon dioxide, which is a waste product of cellular metabolism, diffuses from the capillaries into the alveoli to be exhaled. In this way, the body gets the oxygen it needs to function properly, while also getting rid of carbon dioxide that would otherwise accumulate and cause harm.

The lungs rely on a complex system of muscles and connective tissues for support. Among them, the diaphragm, a muscle shaped like a dome located at the base of the lungs, plays a vital role in breathing. When the diaphragm contracts, it flattens and moves downwards, creating a vacuum in the lungs that allows air to be drawn in. Conversely, when the diaphragm relaxes, it moves upwards, pushing the air out of the lungs.

In addition to the diaphragm, other muscles in the chest and abdomen, such as the intercostal muscles, also assist in the breathing process. These muscles help to expand and contract the chest cavity, allowing for the movement of air in and out of the lungs.

The lungs are protected by several defense mechanisms to prevent infection and maintain their function. The respiratory system produces mucus, a sticky substance that traps foreign particles and bacteria. Tiny, hair-like structures called cilia line the airways and help to move the mucus and trapped particles out of the lungs.

In a healthy individual, the lungs are elastic and can expand and contract easily. This allows for efficient gas exchange and normal breathing. However, in individuals with emphysema, the structure and function of the lungs are significantly compromised.

Emphysema is a chronic lung condition characterized by the destruction of the alveoli and the surrounding lung tissue. Over time, exposure to irritants, such as cigarette smoke or air pollution, leads to inflammation and damage to the delicate walls of the alveoli. This damage reduces the elasticity of the lungs and impairs their ability to effectively exchange oxygen and carbon dioxide.

As emphysema progresses, the air sacs lose their shape and become enlarged. This leads to the formation of large air spaces called bullae, which can further compromise lung function. The destruction of lung tissue also reduces the surface area available for gas exchange, resulting in decreased oxygen levels in the blood and increased carbon dioxide levels.

How Emphysema Affects the Lungs

Emphysema is a chronic lung condition that primarily affects the air sacs, known as alveoli, in the lungs. These tiny air sacs are responsible for the exchange of oxygen and carbon dioxide during the process of breathing. In a healthy lung, the alveoli are elastic and expand and contract easily. However, in emphysema, the walls of the alveoli become damaged and lose their elasticity, leading to a range of respiratory problems.

The main cause of emphysema is long-term exposure to irritants, particularly cigarette smoke. When a person inhales smoke, harmful chemicals and toxins are deposited in the lungs. Over time, these substances cause inflammation and damage to the delicate tissues of the alveoli. As a result, the walls of the air sacs lose their elasticity and become stretched out, leading to the formation of large, irregular air spaces.

The damage to the alveoli in emphysema has several significant effects on lung function. Firstly, the loss of elasticity makes it difficult for the lungs to fully exhale air. This leads to air becoming trapped in the lungs, causing them to overinflate. As a result, the lungs become hyperinflated, which can lead to a barrel-shaped chest appearance.

Secondly, the destruction of the alveoli reduces the surface area available for gas exchange. With fewer functional air sacs, the lungs are less efficient at taking in oxygen and removing carbon dioxide. This can result in a decrease in oxygen levels in the blood and an increase in carbon dioxide levels, leading to a condition known as respiratory failure.

The reduced ability of the lungs to exchange gases also leads to shortness of breath, a hallmark symptom of emphysema. As the damaged alveoli struggle to deliver oxygen to the bloodstream, the body may not receive an adequate supply of oxygen. This can cause feelings of breathlessness, especially during physical exertion or even at rest in severe cases.

In addition to these primary effects, emphysema can also impact other structures within the lungs. The destruction of the alveolar walls can weaken the support structures of the airways, leading to their collapse and narrowing. This can further obstruct the flow of air in and out of the lungs, exacerbating breathing difficulties.

Furthermore, the chronic inflammation and damage caused by emphysema can trigger an immune response in the lungs. This immune response can lead to the production of excess mucus, which can clog the airways and make breathing even more challenging. The combination of narrowed airways and excessive mucus production can result in frequent respiratory infections, such as bronchitis or pneumonia.

As emphysema progresses, the damage to the lungs becomes irreversible. The destruction of the alveoli is a progressive process, and once the damage is done, it cannot be reversed. However, early diagnosis and appropriate management can help slow down the progression of the disease and alleviate symptoms.

Individuals with emphysema need to understand how the condition affects their lungs. By understanding the underlying mechanisms of the disease, individuals can make informed decisions about their treatment and lifestyle choices. With proper management and support, individuals with emphysema can lead fulfilling lives and minimize the impact of the disease on their lung function.

Types of Emphysema

Emphysema is a chronic lung condition that is characterized by the destruction of the air sacs in the lungs, known as alveoli. This destruction leads to the formation of large air spaces, which reduces the surface area available for oxygen exchange. While emphysema is generally classified as a single condition, different types of emphysema can occur based on various factors.

1. Centrilobular Emphysema

Centrilobular emphysema is the most common type of emphysema and is typically associated with cigarette smoking. It primarily affects the upper lobes of the lungs and is characterized by the destruction of the respiratory bronchioles, which are the small airways that branch off from the bronchi. Over time, the damage spreads to the surrounding alveoli, leading to the formation of larger air spaces. Centrilobular emphysema is often seen in individuals with a long history of smoking and is more prevalent in older adults.

2. Panlobular Emphysema

Panlobular emphysema, also known as panacinar emphysema, is less common than centrilobular emphysema but tends to be more severe. It affects the entire acinus, which includes the respiratory bronchioles, alveolar ducts, and alveoli. Panlobular emphysema is often associated with a genetic condition called alpha-1 antitrypsin deficiency, where the body lacks a protein that protects the lungs from damage. This type of emphysema is typically seen in younger individuals and can progress rapidly.

3. Paraseptal Emphysema

Paraseptal emphysema, also known as distal acinar emphysema, is characterized by the destruction of the alveoli adjacent to the pleura, which is the thin membrane that covers the lungs. It often occurs in the lower lobes of the lungs and is commonly seen in individuals with a history of smoking. Paraseptal emphysema is usually asymptomatic and may not cause significant breathing difficulties unless it progresses or is accompanied by other types of emphysema.

4. Irregular Emphysema

Irregular emphysema is a less common type of emphysema that is characterized by irregularly shaped areas of lung tissue destruction. It can occur in various parts of the lungs and is often associated with underlying lung diseases such as bronchiectasis or fibrosis. Irregular emphysema can cause localized areas of air trapping and may lead to complications such as pneumothorax (collapsed lung) or respiratory infections.

5. Bullous Emphysema

Bullous emphysema is characterized by the formation of large air spaces called bullae. These bullae are thin-walled and can vary in size, ranging from a few centimeters to several centimeters in diameter. Bullous emphysema is often associated with severe emphysema and can cause significant breathing difficulties. It is commonly seen in individuals with a long history of smoking and may require surgical intervention to remove the bullae and improve lung function.

6. Combined Emphysema

Combined emphysema refers to a combination of different types of emphysema occurring in the same individual. For example, a person may have both centrilobular and panlobular emphysema or a combination of centrilobular and paraseptal emphysema. Combined emphysema can lead to more severe symptoms and complications compared to a single type of emphysema.

It is important to note that the classification of emphysema types is not always clear-cut, and there can be overlap between different types. Additionally, individuals with emphysema may exhibit characteristics of multiple types simultaneously. The specific type of emphysema a person has can influence the progression of the disease, the severity of symptoms, and the treatment options available.

Understanding the different types of emphysema can help healthcare professionals tailor treatment plans to individual patients and provide appropriate management strategies. Individuals with emphysema need to work closely with their healthcare team to determine the most effective approach for their specific condition.

Complications and Associated Conditions

Emphysema is a chronic lung condition that can lead to various complications and associated conditions. While the primary characteristic of emphysema is the destruction of the air sacs in the lungs, the effects of this condition can extend beyond the respiratory system. Understanding these complications and associated conditions is crucial for effectively managing emphysema and improving overall health outcomes.

1. Respiratory Complications

- **Chronic Bronchitis:** Emphysema often coexists with chronic bronchitis, a condition characterized by inflammation and narrowing of the airways. The combination of emphysema and chronic bronchitis is known as chronic obstructive pulmonary disease (COPD). Chronic bronchitis can cause excessive mucus production, leading to persistent coughing and difficulty breathing.

- **Pneumonia:** People with emphysema are at an increased risk of developing pneumonia. The damaged air sacs in the lungs make it easier for bacteria or viruses to invade and cause infection. Pneumonia can further compromise lung function and worsen respiratory symptoms.

- **Pulmonary Hypertension:** Emphysema can lead to pulmonary hypertension, a condition characterized by high blood pressure in the arteries of the lungs.

The destruction of lung tissue and the resulting loss of functional capillaries can increase the resistance to blood flow in the lungs, leading to elevated blood pressure. Pulmonary hypertension can strain the heart and impair its ability to pump blood efficiently.

- **Respiratory Failure:** In severe cases of emphysema, the lungs may become so damaged that they fail to provide adequate oxygen to the body and remove carbon dioxide effectively. This can result in respiratory failure, a life-threatening condition that requires immediate medical intervention.

2. Cardiovascular Complications

- **Coronary Artery Disease:** Emphysema is associated with an increased risk of developing coronary artery disease (CAD). CAD occurs when the blood vessels that supply the heart with oxygen and nutrients become narrowed or blocked due to the buildup of plaque. The combination of emphysema and CAD can significantly impact heart health and increase the risk of heart attacks.

- **Heart Failure:** The strain placed on the heart due to emphysema and associated conditions can lead to heart failure. Heart failure occurs when the heart is unable to pump blood efficiently, resulting in fluid buildup in the lungs and other parts of the body. Symptoms of heart failure include shortness of breath, fatigue, and swelling in the legs and ankles.

- **Arrhythmias:** Emphysema can disrupt the normal electrical signals in the heart, leading to irregular heart rhythms, or arrhythmias. Arrhythmias can cause palpitations, dizziness, and fainting. Individuals with emphysema need to monitor their heart health and seek medical attention if they experience any abnormal heart rhythms.

3. Other Complications

- **Weight Loss and Malnutrition:** The increased effort required to breathe by individuals with emphysema can lead to a higher calorie expenditure. This, combined with a reduced appetite due to breathlessness and fatigue, can result in weight loss and malnutrition. Individuals with emphysema must maintain a healthy diet and ensure they are receiving adequate nutrition.

- **Depression and Anxiety:** Living with a chronic condition like emphysema can take a toll on mental and emotional well-being. Many individuals with emphysema experience symptoms of depression and anxiety. It is important to address these psychological aspects of the condition and seek support from healthcare professionals or support groups.

- **Osteoporosis:** Emphysema and the use of certain medications for its treatment can increase the risk of developing osteoporosis, a condition characterized by weak and brittle bones. Regular exercise, a balanced diet, and appropriate supplementation can help maintain bone health in individuals with emphysema.

- **Sleep Disorders:** Emphysema can disrupt normal sleep patterns and lead to sleep disorders such as sleep apnea. Sleep apnea is a condition where breathing repeatedly stops and starts during sleep. It can further contribute to fatigue and worsen respiratory symptoms during the day.

Understanding these complications and associated conditions is essential for individuals with emphysema and their healthcare providers. By recognizing and addressing these potential issues, individuals can take proactive steps to manage their condition effectively and improve their overall quality of life. Regular medical check-ups, adherence to treatment plans, and a healthy lifestyle can help minimize the impact of these complications and associated conditions on individuals with emphysema.

Chapter 3

Managing Emphysema

Lifestyle Changes for Better Lung Health

Making lifestyle changes is an essential part of managing emphysema and improving lung health. By adopting healthy habits and avoiding certain triggers, individuals with emphysema can reduce symptoms, slow down the progression of the disease, and enhance their overall quality of life.

1. Quit Smoking

If you are a smoker and have been diagnosed with emphysema, quitting smoking is the most crucial lifestyle change you can make. Smoking is the leading cause of emphysema, and continuing to smoke will only worsen the condition. Quitting smoking can help slow down the progression of the disease, improve lung function, and reduce the risk of complications. It is never too late to quit smoking, and there are various resources available to assist you in this process, such as nicotine replacement therapy, medications, and support groups.

2. Avoid Secondhand Smoke and Environmental Pollutants

In addition to quitting smoking, it is important to avoid exposure to secondhand smoke and environmental pollutants. Secondhand smoke can be just as harmful as smoking itself, so it is crucial to stay away from areas where smoking is allowed. Environmental pollutants, such as air pollution and chemical fumes, can also aggravate emphysema symptoms. If you live in an area with poor air quality, consider using air purifiers in your home and avoiding outdoor activities during times of high pollution.

3. Maintain a Healthy Weight

Maintaining a healthy weight is important for individuals with emphysema. Excess weight can put additional strain on the lungs and make breathing more difficult. On the other hand, being underweight can weaken the respiratory muscles and make it harder to fight off infections. It is recommended to work with a healthcare professional or a registered dietitian to develop a balanced eating plan that meets your nutritional needs and helps you maintain a healthy weight.

4. Exercise Regularly

Regular exercise is beneficial for individuals with emphysema as it can improve lung function, increase stamina, and enhance overall fitness. Engaging in aerobic exercises, such as walking, swimming, or cycling, can help strengthen the respiratory muscles and improve the efficiency of oxygen uptake. It is important to start slowly and gradually increase the intensity and duration of exercise. Consult with your healthcare provider before starting any exercise program to ensure it is safe and appropriate for your condition.

5. Practice Breathing Techniques

Learning and practicing breathing techniques can help individuals with emphysema manage breathlessness and improve lung function. Techniques such as pursed-lip breathing and diaphragmatic breathing can help slow down breathing, reduce shortness of breath, and increase oxygen intake. These techniques can be learned through pulmonary rehabilitation programs or with the guidance of a respiratory therapist.

6. Manage Stress

Stress can worsen emphysema symptoms and make it harder to breathe. Finding effective ways to manage stress is crucial for individuals with emphysema. Engaging in relaxation techniques, such as deep breathing exercises, meditation, or yoga, can help reduce stress and promote a sense of calm. It is also important to prioritize self-care, engage in activities that bring joy and relaxation, and seek support from friends, family, or support groups.

7. Get Vaccinated

Individuals with emphysema are at a higher risk of developing respiratory infections, which can further damage the lungs. Getting vaccinated against influenza and pneumonia is essential for preventing these infections. Consult with your healthcare provider to ensure you are up to date with your vaccinations and discuss any additional vaccines that may be recommended for your specific situation.

8. Avoid Respiratory Irritants

Certain substances can irritate the lungs and worsen emphysema symptoms. It is important to avoid exposure to respiratory irritants such as strong chemicals, dust, fumes, and allergens. If you work in an environment where you are exposed to these irritants, consider wearing protective masks or exploring alternative work arrangements.

9. Stay Hydrated

Drinking an adequate amount of water is important for individuals with emphysema. Staying hydrated helps keep the mucus in the airways thin and easier to cough up, reducing the risk of infections. Aim to drink at least 8 cups of water per day, unless otherwise advised by your healthcare provider.

10. Follow a Healthy Diet

Eating a nutritious diet can support overall health and lung function. Include a variety of fruits, vegetables, whole grains, lean proteins, and healthy fats in your diet. Avoid foods that can cause bloating or gas, as they can put pressure on the diaphragm and make breathing more difficult. It is also important to limit your intake of sodium, as it can contribute to fluid retention and worsen breathing difficulties.

By implementing these lifestyle changes, individuals with emphysema can take an active role in managing their condition and improving their lung health. It is important to work closely with healthcare professionals to develop a personalized plan that addresses your specific needs and goals. Remember, small changes can make a big difference in managing emphysema and enhancing your overall well-being.

Medications for Emphysema

Medications play a crucial role in the management of emphysema. They can help alleviate symptoms, reduce inflammation, and improve lung function. In this section, we will explore the different types of medications commonly used to treat emphysema and how they work.

1. Bronchodilators

Bronchodilators are a class of medications that relax the muscles around the airways, allowing them to open up and improve airflow. They are often the first line of treatment for emphysema and are available in various forms, including inhalers, nebulizers, and pills.

Short-acting bronchodilators provide quick relief and are used as rescue medications during sudden episodes of breathlessness. They work rapidly to open up the airways and provide immediate relief. Examples of short-acting bronchodilators include albuterol (Ventolin) and ipratropium (Atrovent).

Long-acting bronchodilators, on the other hand, provide sustained relief and are used regularly to prevent symptoms and improve lung function. They are typically prescribed in combination with other medications. Examples of long-acting bronchodilators include tiotropium (Spiriva) and formoterol (Foradil).

2. Inhaled Corticosteroids

Inhaled corticosteroids are anti-inflammatory medications that help reduce airway inflammation and prevent exacerbations in emphysema. They are often used in combination with bronchodilators to provide comprehensive treatment. Inhaled corticosteroids are available as inhalers and are typically used daily.

Commonly prescribed inhaled corticosteroids include fluticasone (Flovent) and budesonide (Pulmicort). It's important to note that these medications are not suitable for everyone and may have side effects, such as oral thrush or hoarseness. Your healthcare provider will determine if inhaled corticosteroids are appropriate for you based on your individual needs and medical history.

3. Combination Medications

Combination medications are a convenient option for individuals with emphysema who require both bronchodilators and inhaled corticosteroids. These medications combine the benefits of both classes of drugs into a single inhaler, simplifying the treatment regimen.

Examples of combination medications include fluticasone/salmeterol (Advair) and budesonide/formoterol (Symbicort). They are typically used regularly to provide long-term symptom control and prevent exacerbations.

4. Antibiotics

In some cases, emphysema can lead to frequent respiratory infections, which can further worsen symptoms and lung function. Antibiotics may be prescribed to treat bacterial infections and prevent complications. Commonly prescribed antibiotics for emphysema include azithromycin and amoxicillin.

It's important to follow the prescribed antibiotic regimen and complete the full course of treatment to effectively eliminate the infection. Additionally, it's crucial to discuss any allergies or potential drug interactions with your healthcare provider before starting antibiotic therapy.

5. Mucolytics

Mucolytics are medications that help thin and loosen mucus in the airways, making it easier to cough up. They can be beneficial for individuals with emphysema who have excessive mucus production and difficulty clearing their airways.

One commonly used mucolytic medication is acetylcysteine (Mucomyst). It is available in both oral and inhalation forms. Mucolytics are typically used regularly to help improve mucus clearance and reduce the risk of respiratory infections.

6. Vaccinations

Vaccinations are an essential part of managing emphysema. They can help prevent respiratory infections, which can be particularly dangerous for individuals with compromised lung function. It is recommended that individuals with emphysema receive the annual influenza vaccine and the pneumococcal vaccine.

The influenza vaccine protects against seasonal flu viruses, while the pneumococcal vaccine helps prevent infections caused by the bacteria Streptococcus pneumoniae. These vaccinations can significantly reduce the risk of respiratory infections and their associated complications.

Pulmonary Rehabilitation

Pulmonary rehabilitation is a comprehensive program designed to help individuals with emphysema improve their lung function, manage their symptoms, and enhance their overall quality of life. It is a multidisciplinary approach that combines exercise training, education, and support to address the physical, emotional, and social aspects of living with emphysema.

The Goals of Pulmonary Rehabilitation

The primary goal of pulmonary rehabilitation is to improve the functional capacity of the lungs and reduce the impact of emphysema on daily activities. This is achieved through a combination of exercise, education, and behavioral interventions. The specific goals of pulmonary rehabilitation may include:

1. **Improving lung function:** Pulmonary rehabilitation aims to enhance lung capacity and efficiency, allowing individuals with emphysema to breathe more easily and efficiently.

2. **Increasing exercise tolerance:** Regular exercise is an essential component of pulmonary rehabilitation. By gradually increasing physical activity, individuals can improve their endurance and ability to perform daily tasks without becoming breathless.

3. **Enhancing quality of life:** Emphysema can significantly impact a person's quality of life.

Pulmonary rehabilitation helps individuals manage their symptoms, reduce anxiety and depression, and improve their overall well-being.

4. **Educating about self-management:** Pulmonary rehabilitation programs provide education on various aspects of emphysema, including medication management, breathing techniques, energy conservation, and coping strategies. This knowledge empowers individuals to take an active role in managing their condition.

Components of Pulmonary Rehabilitation

Pulmonary rehabilitation programs typically consist of the following components:

1. **Exercise training:** Exercise is a crucial part of pulmonary rehabilitation. It includes aerobic exercises, such as walking or cycling, to improve cardiovascular fitness, as well as strength training exercises to enhance muscle strength and endurance. Exercise programs are tailored to the individual's abilities and gradually progress over time.

2. **Education and self-management:** Education sessions cover a wide range of topics related to

emphysema, including the disease process, medication management, breathing techniques, nutrition, and stress management. These sessions aim to provide individuals with the knowledge and skills necessary to manage their condition effectively.

3. **Breathing exercises:** Pulmonary rehabilitation includes teaching individuals various breathing techniques to improve lung function and reduce breathlessness. Techniques such as pursed-lip breathing and diaphragmatic breathing can help individuals control their breathing and reduce the work of breathing.

4. **Psychological support:** Living with emphysema can be emotionally challenging. Pulmonary rehabilitation programs often include counseling or support groups to help individuals cope with anxiety, depression, and other emotional issues related to their condition.

5. **Nutritional counseling:** Good nutrition is essential for individuals with emphysema to maintain their overall health and energy levels. Pulmonary rehabilitation programs may include sessions with a

registered dietitian, who can provide guidance on healthy eating habits and weight management.

Benefits of Pulmonary Rehabilitation

Participating in a pulmonary rehabilitation program can offer numerous benefits for individuals with emphysema. Some of the key benefits include:

1. **Improved lung function:** Regular exercise and breathing techniques can help improve lung capacity and efficiency, allowing individuals to breathe more easily and reduce breathlessness.
2. **Increased exercise tolerance:** Through structured exercise programs, individuals can gradually increase their exercise tolerance and perform daily activities with less effort.
3. **Enhanced quality of life:** Pulmonary rehabilitation can improve overall well-being by reducing symptoms, increasing energy levels, and improving emotional well-being.
4. **Better self-management:** Education and self-management strategies provided in pulmonary rehabilitation programs empower individuals to take control of their condition and make informed decisions about their health.

5. **Reduced hospitalizations:** Studies have shown that individuals who participate in pulmonary rehabilitation programs have fewer hospitalizations and emergency room visits related to their emphysema.

How to Access Pulmonary Rehabilitation

Pulmonary rehabilitation programs are typically offered in specialized clinics or hospitals. To access pulmonary rehabilitation, individuals should consult their healthcare provider, who can provide a referral to a program in their area. Insurance coverage for pulmonary rehabilitation varies, so it is essential to check with the insurance provider regarding coverage and any associated costs.

Surgical Options

In some cases, surgical intervention may be necessary to manage emphysema. Surgical options for emphysema aim to improve lung function, reduce symptoms, and enhance the overall quality of life for individuals with this condition. It is important to note that not all individuals with emphysema will require surgery, and the decision to undergo a surgical procedure should be made in consultation with a healthcare professional.

Lung Volume Reduction Surgery (LVRS)

Lung volume reduction surgery (LVRS) is a procedure that involves removing damaged lung tissue to improve lung function. This surgery is typically recommended for individuals with severe emphysema who have significant airflow limitations and symptoms that are not adequately controlled with other treatments.

During the procedure, the surgeon removes small sections of damaged lung tissue, allowing the remaining healthier lung tissue to expand and function more efficiently. This can help improve breathing and reduce symptoms such as shortness of breath.

LVRS can be performed through different approaches, including open surgery or minimally invasive techniques such as video-assisted thoracoscopic surgery (VATS). VATS involves making small incisions and using a video camera and specialized instruments to perform the surgery. Minimally invasive techniques generally result in shorter hospital stays, faster recovery times, and reduced post-operative pain compared to open surgery.

It is important to note that LVRS is not suitable for everyone with emphysema. The procedure is typically recommended for individuals who have predominantly upper lobe emphysema and good exercise capacity. A thorough evaluation by a healthcare professional is necessary to determine if an individual is a suitable candidate for LVRS.

Lung Transplantation

For individuals with end-stage emphysema who have severe lung damage and impaired lung function, lung transplantation may be considered as a treatment option. Lung transplantation involves replacing one or both diseased lungs with healthy lungs from a donor.

The decision to undergo lung transplantation is complex and requires careful consideration. It is typically reserved for individuals who have exhausted all other treatment options and have a poor prognosis without transplantation. The evaluation process for lung transplantation involves a comprehensive assessment of the individual's overall health, lung function, and ability to tolerate the surgery and post-transplant medications.

Lung transplantation can significantly improve lung function and quality of life for individuals with end-stage emphysema. However, it is important to note that the procedure carries risks and complications, and lifelong immunosuppressive medications are required to prevent organ rejection.

Bullectomy

A bullectomy is a surgical procedure that involves removing large air spaces called bullae that form in the lungs of individuals with emphysema. Bullae are abnormal air-filled spaces that develop when the walls of the air sacs in the lungs are destroyed, leading to the formation of large air pockets.

Bullae can compress the surrounding healthy lung tissue, impairing lung function and causing symptoms such as shortness of breath. By removing the bullae, the remaining lung tissue can function more effectively, improving breathing and reducing symptoms.

Bullectomy can be performed through open surgery or minimally invasive techniques such as VATS. The choice of approach depends on various factors, including the size and location of the bullae and the individual's overall health.

It is important to note that not all individuals with emphysema will have bullae, and not all bullae require surgical intervention. The decision to undergo a bullectomy is based on the individual's symptoms, lung function, and the size and location of the bullae.

Lung Volume Reduction Coils

Lung volume reduction coils are a minimally invasive treatment option for individuals with emphysema. This procedure involves placing small coils into the lungs to reduce hyperinflation and improve lung function.

The coils work by compressing the damaged lung tissue, allowing the healthier lung tissue to expand and function more efficiently. This can help improve breathing and reduce symptoms such as shortness of breath.

Lung volume reduction coils are typically placed using a bronchoscope, a thin, flexible tube that is inserted through the mouth or nose and into the airways. The coils are then deployed into the lungs, where they remain in place to provide ongoing support to the lung tissue.

This procedure is less invasive than traditional surgical options and can be performed on an outpatient basis. However, not all individuals with emphysema are suitable candidates for lung volume reduction coils, and a thorough evaluation by a healthcare professional is necessary to determine if this procedure is appropriate.

Other Surgical Procedures

In addition to the surgical options mentioned above, other less common surgical procedures may be considered for individuals with emphysema. These include lung transplantation with volume reduction, which combines lung transplantation with the removal of damaged lung tissue, and bronchoscopic lung volume reduction, which involves using special devices to block off or collapse damaged airways.

These procedures are typically reserved for individuals who have specific characteristics or circumstances that make them suitable candidates. The decision to undergo these procedures should be made in consultation with a healthcare professional who can assess the individual's specific needs and circumstances.

Oxygen Therapy

Oxygen therapy is a common treatment option for individuals with emphysema. It involves the use of supplemental oxygen to help improve oxygen levels in the blood and alleviate symptoms associated with low oxygen levels. This section will provide an overview of oxygen therapy, including its benefits, different delivery methods, and considerations for its use.

Benefits of Oxygen Therapy

Oxygen therapy can provide several benefits for individuals with emphysema. The primary goal of this treatment is to increase the oxygen levels in the blood, which can help improve overall health and well-being. Some of the key benefits of oxygen therapy include:

1. **Relief of breathlessness:** One of the most significant benefits of oxygen therapy is its ability to relieve breathlessness, a common symptom of emphysema. By increasing oxygen levels, it can help reduce the feeling of shortness of breath and improve the individual's ability to perform daily activities.

2. **Improved exercise tolerance:** Emphysema can limit an individual's ability to engage in physical activity due to breathlessness. Oxygen therapy can enhance exercise tolerance by providing the necessary oxygen to the muscles, allowing individuals to engage in physical activity for longer durations.

3. **Enhanced cognitive function:** Low oxygen levels in the blood can affect cognitive function, leading to difficulties in concentration and memory. Oxygen

therapy can help improve cognitive function by increasing oxygen supply to the brain.

4. **Better sleep quality:** Many individuals with emphysema experience sleep disturbances due to low oxygen levels. Oxygen therapy can improve sleep quality by ensuring adequate oxygen supply during sleep, leading to better rest and overall well-being.

Delivery Methods

There are different delivery methods available for oxygen therapy, and the choice depends on the individual's needs and preferences. The most common delivery methods include:

1. **Oxygen concentrators:** Oxygen concentrators are devices that extract oxygen from the surrounding air and deliver it to the individual through a nasal cannula or mask. They are portable and can be used at home or while traveling.

2. **Compressed oxygen cylinders:** Compressed oxygen cylinders contain oxygen in compressed form and are available in various sizes. They are typically used for individuals who require higher flow rates or need to be more mobile.

3. **Liquid oxygen systems:** Liquid oxygen systems store oxygen in a liquid form, which is then converted to a gas for inhalation. These systems are suitable for individuals who require higher flow rates and need to be more mobile.

4. **Oxygen-conserving devices:** Oxygen-conserving devices are designed to optimize the use of oxygen by delivering it only during inhalation, conserving oxygen, and extending the duration of use.

The choice of delivery method will depend on factors such as the individual's oxygen requirements, lifestyle, and mobility.

Considerations for Oxygen Therapy

While oxygen therapy can be highly beneficial for individuals with emphysema, there are some considerations to keep in mind:

1. **Prescription and monitoring:** Oxygen therapy should be prescribed by a healthcare professional based on the individual's oxygen saturation levels and specific needs. Regular monitoring of oxygen levels is essential to ensure the therapy is effective and adjusted as necessary.

2. **Safety precautions:** Oxygen is a highly flammable substance, and certain safety precautions should be followed when using oxygen therapy. This includes keeping oxygen equipment away from open flames, avoiding smoking or using flammable materials near oxygen, and ensuring proper ventilation in the room.

3. **Maintenance and cleaning:** Regular maintenance and cleaning of oxygen equipment are necessary to ensure its proper functioning and prevent infections. It is important to follow the manufacturer's instructions for cleaning and replacing equipment components.

4. **Travel considerations:** Individuals who require oxygen therapy may need to make special arrangements when traveling, such as notifying airlines or arranging for portable oxygen concentrators. It is important to plan ahead and ensure a sufficient supply of oxygen during the journey.

Oxygen Therapy and Lifestyle

Oxygen therapy can significantly improve the quality of life for individuals with emphysema, but it may require some adjustments to daily routines and activities. Here are some lifestyle considerations when using oxygen therapy:

1. **Mobility:** Depending on the delivery method, individuals may need to carry portable oxygen equipment with them. This may require using a wheeled cart or backpack to transport the equipment, ensuring mobility while maintaining a sufficient oxygen supply.

2. **Home modifications:** Individuals using oxygen therapy at home may need to make certain modifications to ensure safety and convenience. This may include rearranging furniture to accommodate oxygen tubing, ensuring proper ventilation, and avoiding potential hazards.

3. **Travel planning:** When planning trips or vacations, individuals using oxygen therapy should consider factors such as the availability of oxygen at their destination, transportation arrangements, and any necessary documentation or permits for traveling with oxygen.

4. **Social activities:** Oxygen therapy should not limit social activities. Individuals can participate in social events, gatherings, and hobbies while using oxygen therapy. It is important to communicate with

friends, family, and caregivers about the need for oxygen and any specific requirements.

Managing Exacerbations

Exacerbations, also known as flare-ups or lung attacks, are episodes of worsening symptoms in individuals with emphysema. These episodes can be triggered by various factors, such as respiratory infections, exposure to irritants, or failure to adhere to treatment plans. Managing exacerbations is crucial to minimize their impact on lung function and overall well-being. In this section, we will discuss strategies for effectively managing exacerbations and reducing their frequency.

Recognizing Exacerbations

The first step in managing exacerbations is to be able to recognize when they occur. It is important to be aware of the signs and symptoms that indicate a worsening of your condition. These may include increased breathlessness, coughing, wheezing, chest tightness, increased sputum production, and changes in the color or consistency of the sputum. If you experience any of these symptoms, it is essential to seek medical attention promptly.

Seeking Medical Care

When you suspect an exacerbation, it is crucial to contact your healthcare provider as soon as possible. They will be able to assess your condition and provide appropriate treatment. In some cases, you may need to visit the emergency department if your symptoms are severe or rapidly worsening. It is important not to delay seeking medical care, as prompt intervention can help prevent further deterioration of lung function.

Treatment Options

The treatment for exacerbations may vary depending on the severity of your symptoms. In mild cases, your healthcare provider may prescribe additional medications, such as bronchodilators or corticosteroids, to help relieve symptoms and reduce inflammation in the airways. They may also recommend increasing the frequency of your existing medications.

In more severe cases, hospitalization may be necessary. This allows for closer monitoring and the administration of supplemental oxygen if needed. During hospitalization, you may receive intravenous medications, such as antibiotics or systemic corticosteroids, to treat any underlying infections or inflammation.

Self-Management Strategies

In addition to medical treatment, several self-management strategies can help you cope with exacerbations and promote recovery. These include:

1. **Rest and conserve energy:** During exacerbations, it is important to conserve your energy and avoid overexertion. Resting allows your body to focus on healing and reduces the strain on your lungs.

2. **Stay hydrated:** Drinking plenty of fluids helps thin the mucus in your airways, making it easier to cough up. It is important to drink water and avoid caffeinated or alcoholic beverages, as they can dehydrate you.

3. **Practice breathing techniques:** Breathing exercises, such as pursed-lip breathing and diaphragmatic breathing, can help improve lung function and reduce breathlessness during exacerbations. Your healthcare provider or a respiratory therapist can teach you these techniques.

4. **Maintain good hygiene:** Practicing good hygiene, such as washing your hands frequently and avoiding close contact with individuals who have respiratory infections, can help reduce the risk of exacerbations caused by infections.

5. **Follow your treatment plan:** It is crucial to adhere to your prescribed treatment plan, including taking medications as directed and using any prescribed inhalers or nebulizers. This will help manage your symptoms and prevent exacerbations.

Prevention of Exacerbations

While it may not be possible to completely prevent exacerbations, there are steps you can take to reduce their frequency and severity. These include:

1. **Avoiding triggers:** Identify and avoid triggers that worsen your symptoms, such as cigarette smoke, air pollution, and respiratory infections. If you are exposed to irritants, consider wearing a mask or taking other protective measures.

2. **Getting vaccinated:** Vaccinations, such as the flu vaccine and the pneumonia vaccine, can help prevent respiratory infections that can trigger exacerbations. It is important to discuss vaccination options with your healthcare provider.

3. **Maintaining good lung health:** Engaging in regular physical activity, practicing deep breathing exercises, and following a healthy diet can help

maintain good lung health and reduce the risk of exacerbations.

4. **Regular follow-up with your healthcare provider:** Regular check-ups with your healthcare provider are important to monitor your lung function and adjust your treatment plan as needed. They can also provide guidance on managing exacerbations and answer any questions or concerns you may have.

Chapter 4

Living with Emphysema

Coping with Breathlessness

One of the most challenging symptoms of emphysema is breathlessness, also known as dyspnea. Breathlessness can be a distressing and frightening experience, as it can make you feel like you are not getting enough air. However, several strategies and techniques can help you cope with breathlessness and improve your quality of life.

Understanding Breathlessness

Breathlessness occurs in emphysema due to the damage to the air sacs in the lungs, which leads to a decrease in the surface area available for oxygen exchange. As a result, the lungs have to work harder to take in oxygen and expel carbon dioxide. This increased effort can cause shortness of breath, especially during physical activity or exertion.

It is important to understand that breathlessness is a common symptom of emphysema and does not necessarily mean that your condition is worsening. It is a natural response of the body to the reduced lung function. By learning how to manage breathlessness, you can regain control over your breathing and reduce the anxiety associated with this symptom.

Breathing Techniques

One of the most effective ways to cope with breathlessness is to practice breathing techniques. These techniques can help you control your breathing and reduce the feeling of breathlessness. Here are a few techniques that you can try:

1. **Pursed-lip breathing:** This technique involves inhaling slowly through your nose and exhaling through pursed lips as if you are blowing out a candle. Pursed-lip breathing helps to slow down your breathing and keeps your airways open for longer, allowing for better oxygen exchange.

2. **Diaphragmatic breathing:** Also known as belly breathing, this technique involves breathing deeply into your diaphragm rather than shallowly into your chest. To practice diaphragmatic breathing, place one hand on your abdomen and the other on your chest. Inhale deeply through your nose, allowing your abdomen to rise, and exhale slowly through your mouth, letting your abdomen fall.

3. **Controlled breathing:** This technique involves consciously controlling the rate and depth of your breaths. You can try inhaling for a count of four, holding your breath for a count of two, and exhaling for a count of four. Repeat this pattern several times until you feel more relaxed and in control of your breathing.

4. **Paced breathing:** Paced breathing involves coordinating your breathing with your physical activity. For example, if you are climbing stairs, try to take a breath in for every step you take and exhale as you climb. This technique helps to synchronize your breathing with your movements and can reduce breathlessness during exertion.

Energy Conservation Techniques

In addition to breathing techniques, energy conservation techniques can also help you manage breathlessness and conserve your energy for activities that are important to you. Here are some strategies to consider:

1. **Plan your activities:** Prioritize your activities and plan them in a way that allows for rest breaks in between. Breaking down tasks into smaller, more

manageable parts can help prevent overexertion and reduce breathlessness.

2. **Use assistive devices:** Consider using assistive devices such as a wheeled cart or a trolley to carry heavy items or a shower chair to conserve energy during bathing. These devices can help reduce the physical effort required for daily tasks and minimize breathlessness.

3. **Pace yourself:** Take breaks and rest when needed. Listen to your body and avoid pushing yourself too hard. Pace yourself throughout the day to avoid becoming overly fatigued and breathless.

4. **Optimize your environment:** Make your living space more comfortable and conducive to breathing. Ensure good ventilation, maintain a comfortable temperature, and minimize exposure to irritants such as smoke, dust, and strong odors.

Psychological Strategies

Breathlessness can be emotionally distressing, and anxiety can exacerbate the sensation of breathlessness. Therefore, it is important to address the psychological aspect of coping with breathlessness. Here are some strategies to consider:

1. **Relaxation techniques:** Practice relaxation techniques such as deep breathing, progressive muscle relaxation, or guided imagery to reduce anxiety and promote a sense of calmness. These techniques can help you relax and manage breathlessness more effectively.

2. **Distraction techniques:** Engage in activities that divert your attention away from breathlessness, such as listening to music, reading a book, or watching a movie. By focusing on something enjoyable or interesting, you can shift your focus away from your breathing and reduce anxiety.

3. **Support and counseling:** Seek support from friends, family, or support groups who understand what you are going through. Consider talking to a counselor or therapist who can provide guidance and help you develop coping strategies for managing breathlessness.

Remember, coping with breathlessness is a process that requires practice and patience. By incorporating these techniques into your daily routine and seeking support when needed, you can improve your ability to manage breathlessness and enhance your overall well-being.

Exercise and Physical Activity

Regular exercise and physical activity play a crucial role in managing emphysema. While it may seem counterintuitive to engage in physical activity when you have a condition that affects your breathing, exercise can improve your lung function, increase your stamina, and enhance your overall quality of life. In this section, we will explore the benefits of exercise for individuals with emphysema and provide practical tips on how to incorporate physical activity into your daily routine.

The Benefits of Exercise for Emphysema

Engaging in regular exercise offers numerous benefits for individuals with emphysema. Here are some of the key advantages:

1. **Improved Lung Function:** Exercise helps to strengthen the muscles involved in breathing, such as the diaphragm and intercostal muscles. As these muscles become stronger, they can assist in expanding and contracting the lungs more efficiently, leading to improved lung function.

2. **Increased Stamina:** Emphysema often causes shortness of breath and fatigue, making even simple tasks challenging. Regular exercise can help build

endurance and increase your stamina, allowing you to perform daily activities with less effort and fatigue.

3. **Enhanced Cardiovascular Health:** Exercise promotes cardiovascular fitness, which is essential for individuals with emphysema. By improving your heart and lung health, exercise can reduce the strain on your respiratory system and improve your overall cardiovascular function.

4. **Weight Management:** Many individuals with emphysema struggle with maintaining a healthy weight. Regular exercise can help you manage your weight by burning calories and increasing your metabolism. Additionally, exercise can help build muscle mass, which can further improve your overall physical strength and endurance.

5. **Mental and Emotional Well-being:** Living with emphysema can be emotionally challenging. Exercise has been shown to release endorphins, which are natural mood boosters. Engaging in physical activity can help reduce stress, anxiety, and depression, improving your mental and emotional well-being.

Types of Exercise for Emphysema

When it comes to exercise for individuals with emphysema, it is important to choose activities that are safe and suitable for your condition. Here are some types of exercise that are generally well-tolerated by individuals with emphysema:

1. **Aerobic Exercise:** Aerobic exercises, such as walking, swimming, cycling, and dancing, are excellent choices for individuals with emphysema. These activities increase your heart rate and breathing rate, improving your cardiovascular fitness and overall endurance. Start with low-impact exercises and gradually increase the intensity and duration as your fitness level improves.

2. **Strength Training:** Strength training exercises help build muscle strength and improve overall physical function. Use light weights or resistance bands to perform exercises targeting major muscle groups, such as the arms, legs, and core. It is important to start with light resistance and gradually increase the intensity to avoid straining your muscles.

3. **Breathing Exercises:** Breathing exercises, such as pursed lip breathing and diaphragmatic breathing, can help improve your lung function and control shortness of breath. These exercises focus on deep,

slow breathing techniques that can be practiced both during exercise and in daily life.

4. **Flexibility and Stretching:** Flexibility exercises, such as yoga and stretching, can help improve your range of motion and reduce muscle stiffness. These exercises can be particularly beneficial for individuals with emphysema, as they can help alleviate muscle tension and improve posture.

Tips for Exercising with Emphysema

Before starting any exercise program, it is important to consult with your healthcare provider, especially if you have any underlying health conditions or concerns. Here are some additional tips to keep in mind when exercising with emphysema:

1. **Start Slowly:** Begin with low-intensity exercises and gradually increase the duration and intensity as your fitness level improves. Listen to your body and take breaks when needed.

2. **Warm Up and Cool Down:** Always start your exercise session with a warm-up to prepare your muscles and joints for activity. Similarly, end your session with a cool-down to gradually lower your heart rate and prevent muscle soreness.

3. **Stay Hydrated:** Drink plenty of water before, during, and after exercise to stay hydrated. Proper hydration is essential for maintaining optimal lung function.

4. **Use Assistive Devices if Needed:** If you require supplemental oxygen, make sure to use it as prescribed during exercise. Additionally, consider using assistive devices such as a walker or cane for added stability and support.

5. **Listen to Your Body:** Pay attention to any signs of discomfort or excessive shortness of breath during exercise. If you experience chest pain, dizziness, or severe shortness of breath, stop exercising and seek medical attention.

6. **Stay Consistent:** Aim for regular exercise sessions, ideally at least three to five times per week. Consistency is key to reaping the long-term benefits of exercise for managing emphysema.

Remember, every individual is unique, and what works for one person may not work for another. It is important to find activities that you enjoy and that are suitable for your fitness level and overall health. With the guidance of your healthcare provider, you can develop an exercise routine that is safe, effective, and tailored to your specific needs and abilities.

Nutrition and Diet

Proper nutrition and a healthy diet play a crucial role in managing emphysema. A well-balanced diet can help improve your overall health, strengthen your immune system, and provide the necessary nutrients to support your lung function. In this section, we will explore the importance of nutrition and provide practical tips on how to maintain a healthy diet while living with emphysema.

The Role of Nutrition in Emphysema

Emphysema is a chronic lung condition that affects the air sacs in the lungs, making it difficult to breathe. This condition can lead to weight loss and muscle wasting due to the increased energy expenditure associated with breathing difficulties. Therefore, it is essential to focus on maintaining a healthy weight and providing your body with the necessary nutrients to support your lung function.

Key Nutrients for Emphysema

1. **Protein:** Protein is essential for repairing and building tissues, including the muscles involved in

breathing. Including lean sources of protein such as poultry, fish, beans, and tofu in your diet can help maintain muscle mass and strength.

2. **Omega-3 Fatty Acids:** Omega-3 fatty acids have anti-inflammatory properties and can help reduce inflammation in the lungs. Foods rich in omega-3 fatty acids include fatty fish like salmon and mackerel, walnuts, flaxseeds, and chia seeds.

3. **Antioxidants:** Antioxidants help protect the body from damage caused by free radicals, which can contribute to lung inflammation. Foods rich in antioxidants include fruits and vegetables, especially those with vibrant colors like berries, spinach, kale, and bell peppers.

4. **Fiber:** A high-fiber diet can help prevent constipation, a common side effect of some medications used to manage emphysema. Whole grains, fruits, vegetables, and legumes are excellent sources of fiber.

5. **Vitamin D:** Vitamin D plays a crucial role in lung health and immune function. Spending time outdoors in the sun and consuming foods fortified with vitamin D, such as fortified dairy products,

fatty fish, and egg yolks, can help maintain adequate levels of this essential vitamin.

Tips for a Healthy Diet

1. **Eat a Variety of Foods:** Aim to include a wide range of nutrient-dense foods in your diet to ensure you are getting all the necessary vitamins and minerals. This includes fruits, vegetables, whole grains, lean proteins, and healthy fats.

2. **Portion Control:** Pay attention to portion sizes to avoid overeating. Use smaller plates and bowls to help control portion sizes and prevent excessive calorie intake.

3. **Stay Hydrated:** Drinking enough water is essential for maintaining proper lung function and preventing dehydration. Aim to drink at least eight glasses of water per day and avoid excessive consumption of sugary drinks and caffeine.

4. **Limit Sodium Intake:** Too much sodium can lead to fluid retention and worsen breathing difficulties. Limit your intake of processed and packaged foods, which are often high in sodium, and opt for fresh, whole foods instead.

5. **Avoid Gas-Producing Foods:** Some foods can cause bloating and gas, which can make breathing more difficult. These foods include beans, lentils, broccoli, cabbage, onions, and carbonated beverages. Experiment with your diet to identify any specific foods that may worsen your symptoms.

6. **Consider Small, Frequent Meals:** Eating smaller, more frequent meals can help prevent feelings of fullness and discomfort, making it easier to breathe. Aim for five to six smaller meals throughout the day instead of three large meals.

7. **Consult a Registered Dietitian:** If you have specific dietary concerns or need personalized guidance, consider consulting a registered dietitian who specializes in respiratory conditions. They can provide tailored advice and help you create a meal plan that suits your individual needs.

Mental and Emotional Well-being

Living with emphysema can be challenging not only physically but also mentally and emotionally. The impact of this chronic lung condition can affect your overall well-being and quality of life. It is important to address the mental and emotional aspects of living with emphysema to effectively manage the condition and maintain a positive outlook. In this section, we will explore the various strategies and techniques that can help you maintain good mental and emotional well-being while living with emphysema.

Understanding the Emotional Impact

Emphysema can have a significant emotional impact on individuals. The physical limitations and challenges associated with the condition can lead to feelings of frustration, anxiety, and even depression. It is important to recognize and acknowledge these emotions to effectively address them.

One of the most common emotional challenges faced by individuals with emphysema is anxiety. The shortness of breath and difficulty breathing can cause individuals to feel anxious and fearful, especially during exacerbations or when engaging in physical activities. It is important to learn techniques to manage anxiety, such as deep breathing exercises, relaxation techniques, and mindfulness practices. These techniques can help calm the mind and reduce anxiety levels.

Depression is another common emotional challenge faced by individuals with emphysema. The chronic nature of the condition, along with the physical limitations it imposes, can lead to feelings of sadness, hopelessness, and a loss of interest in activities. It is important to seek support from healthcare professionals, friends, and family members if you are experiencing symptoms of depression. They can provide guidance and support, and they may recommend therapy or medication to help manage these symptoms.

Building a Support System

Having a strong support system is crucial for maintaining good mental and emotional well-being while living with emphysema. Surrounding yourself with understanding and supportive individuals can provide a sense of comfort and encouragement. This support system can include family members, friends, healthcare professionals, and support groups.

Family members and close friends can play a vital role in providing emotional support. They can offer a listening ear, help with daily tasks, and provide encouragement during difficult times. It is important to communicate openly with your loved ones about your feelings and needs and to let them know how they can best support you.

Healthcare professionals, such as your primary care physician or pulmonologist, can also provide valuable support and guidance. They can help you understand your condition better, provide treatment options, and refer you to other healthcare professionals or support groups.

Support groups specifically for individuals with emphysema can be a great source of emotional support. These groups provide a safe space to share experiences, learn from others, and gain a sense of belonging. Support groups can be found in local communities, hospitals, or online platforms. Connecting with others who are going through similar experiences can help reduce feelings of isolation and provide a sense of camaraderie.

Managing Stress

Stress can exacerbate the symptoms of emphysema and negatively impact your mental and emotional well-being. Learning effective stress management techniques can help you cope with the challenges of living with emphysema.

One of the most effective ways to manage stress is through relaxation techniques. Deep breathing exercises, progressive muscle relaxation, and guided imagery are all techniques that can help calm the mind and reduce stress levels. These techniques can be practiced daily or during times of increased stress.

Engaging in activities that you enjoy and that help you relax can also be beneficial for managing stress. This can include hobbies like listening to music, reading, or spending time in nature. Finding activities that bring you joy and help you unwind can provide a much-needed break from the challenges of living with emphysema.

Seeking Professional Help

If you find that your mental and emotional well-being is significantly impacted by emphysema, it may be beneficial to seek professional help. Mental health professionals, such as psychologists or therapists, can provide guidance and support in managing the emotional challenges associated with the condition.

Therapy can help you develop coping strategies, improve your emotional resilience, and address any underlying mental health conditions, such as anxiety or depression. Cognitive-behavioral therapy (CBT) is a commonly used therapeutic approach that can help individuals with emphysema develop healthier thought patterns and coping mechanisms. In some cases, medication may be prescribed to help manage symptoms of anxiety or depression.

Chapter 5

Support and Resources

Support Groups and Organizations

Living with emphysema can be challenging, both physically and emotionally. It is important to remember that you are not alone on this journey. There are numerous support groups and organizations dedicated to providing assistance, resources, and a sense of community for individuals with emphysema and their caregivers.

These groups can offer valuable support, education, and a platform for sharing experiences and coping strategies. In this section, we will explore the benefits of joining support groups and provide a list of reputable organizations that can help you navigate your emphysema journey.

Benefits of Support Groups

Support groups play a crucial role in the management of emphysema. They offer a safe and understanding environment where individuals can connect with others who are facing similar challenges. Here are some of the benefits of joining a support group:

1. **Emotional Support:** Support groups provide a space for individuals to express their feelings, fears, and frustrations. Sharing experiences with others who understand can help alleviate feelings of isolation and provide emotional support.

2. **Information and Education:** Support groups often invite healthcare professionals to speak on various topics related to emphysema. These sessions can provide valuable information about the latest treatments, coping strategies, and self-care techniques.

3. **Practical Advice:** Support groups offer a platform for members to share practical tips and advice on managing daily activities, such as breathing exercises, energy conservation techniques, and navigating healthcare systems.

4. **Sense of Community:** Joining a support group allows individuals to connect with others who are going through similar experiences. This sense of community can provide a much-needed source of encouragement, motivation, and understanding.

5. **Caregiver Support:** Support groups are not only beneficial for individuals with emphysema but also for their caregivers. Caregivers can connect with others who are in similar roles, share their challenges, and learn from each other's experiences.

Reputable Support Groups and Organizations

Here is a list of reputable support groups and organizations that focus on emphysema:

1. **American Lung Association:** The American Lung Association offers a variety of resources and support for individuals with emphysema. They provide educational materials, online support communities, and information on local support groups.

2. **COPD Foundation:** The COPD Foundation is dedicated to improving the lives of individuals with chronic obstructive pulmonary disease (COPD), including emphysema. They offer an online community, educational materials, and resources for patients and caregivers.

3. **Better Breathers Club:** The Better Breathers Club is a program developed by the American Lung Association. It provides support and education for

individuals with lung diseases, including emphysema. These clubs often meet in person and offer a supportive environment for sharing experiences and learning from healthcare professionals.

4. **Alpha-1 Foundation:** The Alpha-1 Foundation focuses on supporting individuals with alpha-1 antitrypsin deficiency, a genetic condition that can lead to emphysema. They provide resources, support groups, and educational materials for individuals and their families.

5. **Pulmonary Education and Research Foundation:** The Pulmonary Education and Research Foundation offers resources, support groups, and educational materials for individuals with various lung diseases, including emphysema. They aim to improve the quality of life for individuals living with these conditions.

6. **Local Hospitals and Medical Centers:** Many hospitals and medical centers have support groups specifically for individuals with lung diseases. These groups often meet regularly and provide a platform for sharing experiences and learning from healthcare professionals.

7. **Online Support Communities:** There are numerous online support communities and forums where individuals with emphysema can connect with others. These communities provide a convenient way to seek support, share experiences, and ask questions.

When considering joining a support group or organization, it is important to research their credibility, reputation, and the services they offer. Reach out to them to inquire about their activities, meeting schedules, and any associated costs.

Remember, support groups and organizations are there to provide assistance and a sense of community. Don't hesitate to reach out and take advantage of the resources available to you. Together, we can navigate the challenges of emphysema and live a fulfilling life.

Financial Assistance and Insurance

Managing emphysema can be a costly endeavor, with medical expenses, medications, and treatments adding up over time. For individuals living with emphysema, it is important to explore financial assistance options and understand how insurance can help cover the costs associated with the condition. In this section, we will discuss various avenues for financial assistance and provide information on insurance coverage for emphysema.

Financial Assistance Programs

1. **Medicare:** Medicare is a federal health insurance program available to individuals aged 65 and older, as well as those with certain disabilities. Medicare Part B covers outpatient services, including doctor visits, medical supplies, and preventive services. Medicare Part D provides prescription drug coverage. It is important to review the specific coverage details and eligibility requirements to determine if Medicare is an option for you.

2. **Medicaid:** Medicaid is a joint federal and state program that provides health coverage to low-income individuals and families. Eligibility requirements vary by state, but Medicaid typically covers a wide range of medical services, including doctor visits, hospital stays, and prescription medications. If you have a low income and limited resources, you may qualify for Medicaid assistance.

3. **Social Security Disability Insurance (SSDI):** SSDI is a federal program that provides financial

assistance to individuals with disabilities who are unable to work. To qualify for SSDI, you must have a disability that meets the Social Security Administration's criteria and have earned enough work credits. If approved, you may be eligible for monthly cash benefits and Medicare coverage after a waiting period.

4. **Supplemental Security Income (SSI):** SSI is a needs-based program that provides financial assistance to individuals with disabilities who have limited income and resources. Unlike SSDI, SSI does not require work credits. If approved for SSI, you may receive monthly cash benefits and may also be eligible for Medicaid coverage.

5. **State Assistance Programs:** Many states offer additional financial assistance programs for individuals with chronic illnesses, including emphysema. These programs may provide coverage for medical services, prescription medications, and other necessary treatments. Contact your state's Department of Health or Social Services to inquire about available programs.

Insurance Coverage

1. **Private Health Insurance:** If you have private health insurance through your employer or purchased it independently, it is important to review your policy to understand what is covered for emphysema. Private insurance plans vary in terms of coverage and cost-sharing requirements. Some plans may cover doctor visits, hospital stays, medications, and pulmonary rehabilitation. Be sure to check if there are any restrictions or limitations on coverage for pre-existing conditions.

2. **Health Insurance Marketplace:** The Health Insurance Marketplace, also known as the Exchange, is a platform where individuals can compare and purchase health insurance plans. Depending on your income, you may qualify for premium tax credits and cost-sharing reductions to help make coverage more affordable. When selecting a plan, consider the specific coverage for emphysema-related services and medications.

3. **COBRA:** If you recently lost your job or experienced a reduction in work hours, you may be eligible for COBRA continuation coverage. COBRA allows you to continue your

employer-sponsored health insurance for a limited time. While COBRA coverage can be expensive, it may provide a temporary solution until you find alternative insurance options.

4. **Veterans Affairs (VA) Benefits:** If you are a veteran, you may be eligible for health care benefits through the Department of Veterans Affairs. The VA provides a range of services for eligible veterans, including diagnosis, treatment, and management of emphysema. Contact your local VA office to determine your eligibility and explore available benefits.

5. **Prescription Assistance Programs:** Many pharmaceutical companies offer patient assistance programs to help individuals afford their medications. These programs provide discounts or free medications to eligible individuals who meet specific income requirements. Contact the pharmaceutical company directly or visit their website to learn more about available programs.

Tips for Navigating Financial Assistance and Insurance

1. **Research and Compare:** Take the time to research and compare different financial assistance programs and insurance options. Each program or plan may have specific eligibility requirements, coverage limitations, and cost-sharing arrangements. By understanding the details, you can make informed decisions about which options are best suited to your needs.

2. **Seek Professional Help:** If you find the process overwhelming or confusing, consider seeking assistance from a healthcare navigator or insurance broker. These professionals can help guide you through the application process, explain your options, and provide personalized advice based on your specific circumstances.

3. **Keep Documentation:** When applying for financial assistance programs or dealing with insurance claims, it is important to keep copies of all relevant documentation. This includes medical records, bills, insurance policies, and correspondence. Having organized records can help streamline the process and provide evidence if any issues arise.

4. **Stay Informed:** Insurance coverage and financial assistance programs can change over time. Stay informed about any updates or changes to your coverage. Review your insurance policy annually and stay in touch with your healthcare provider to ensure you are aware of any new programs or resources that may become available.

Remember, financial assistance and insurance coverage can greatly alleviate the financial burden of managing emphysema. Take the time to explore your options, ask questions, and seek assistance when needed. With the right support, you can focus on managing your condition and improving your quality of life.

Tips for Caregivers

Taking care of someone with emphysema can be a challenging and demanding task. As a caregiver, it is important to understand the needs and limitations of the person you are caring for. This section provides some helpful tips for caregivers to ensure the well-being and comfort of their loved ones with emphysema.

1. **Educate Yourself:** One of the most important things you can do as a caregiver is to educate

yourself about emphysema. Learn about the causes, symptoms, and treatment options for the condition. Understanding the disease will help you provide better care and support for your loved one. Stay updated with the latest research and advancements in emphysema treatment to ensure you are well-informed.

2. **Create a Safe and Comfortable Environment:** Emphysema can make it difficult for individuals to breathe, so it is crucial to create a safe and comfortable environment for them. Ensure that the living space is well-ventilated and free from irritants such as smoke, dust, and strong odors. Keep the home clean and clutter-free to minimize the risk of falls and accidents. Consider installing handrails and grab bars in the bathroom and other areas where support may be needed.

3. **Assist with Medication Management:** Help your loved one with emphysema manage their medications effectively. Create a medication schedule and ensure that they take their medications as prescribed. Set up reminders or use pill organizers to help them stay on track. Keep a record of their medications, including dosages and any side

effects they may experience. Regularly check the medication supply and refill prescriptions on time.

4. **Encourage a Healthy Lifestyle:** Promote a healthy lifestyle for your loved one with emphysema. Encourage them to quit smoking if they haven't already, as smoking can worsen the symptoms of emphysema. Help them follow a nutritious diet that includes plenty of fruits, vegetables, whole grains, and lean proteins. Encourage regular exercise within their capabilities, such as walking or gentle stretching exercises. Ensure they get enough rest and sleep to support their overall well-being.

5. **Provide Emotional Support:** Living with emphysema can be emotionally challenging for both the individual and their caregiver. Be a source of emotional support for your loved one. Listen to their concerns and fears without judgment. Offer reassurance and encouragement. Help them find ways to cope with stress and anxiety, such as practicing relaxation techniques or engaging in enjoyable activities. Consider seeking professional counseling or support groups to help them navigate their emotions.

6. **Assist with Daily Activities:** Emphysema can make everyday tasks more difficult for individuals. Offer assistance with activities such as cooking, cleaning, and personal hygiene. Help them conserve energy by organizing tasks and breaking them down into smaller, manageable steps. Consider using assistive devices such as reachers or shower chairs to make daily activities easier and safer. Encourage independence while being mindful of their limitations.

7. **Monitor Symptoms and Communicate with Healthcare Providers:** As a caregiver, it is important to monitor the symptoms of emphysema and communicate any changes or concerns to healthcare providers. Keep track of any new or worsening symptoms, such as increased breathlessness or coughing. Report any changes in appetite, sleep patterns, or mood. Attend medical appointments with your loved one and ask questions to ensure a clear understanding of their condition and treatment plan.

8. **Seek Respite and Support for Yourself:** Caring for someone with emphysema can be physically and emotionally draining. It is essential to take care of

yourself as well. Seek respite care or ask for help from family members or friends to give yourself a break. Join support groups or seek counseling to connect with other caregivers who can provide understanding and guidance. Remember to prioritize self-care and engage in activities that bring you joy and relaxation.

9. **Be Prepared for Emergencies:** Emphysema can sometimes lead to exacerbations or flare-ups that require immediate medical attention. As a caregiver, it is important to be prepared for emergencies. Keep a list of emergency contact numbers, including the healthcare provider and local emergency services. Familiarize yourself with the signs of a severe exacerbation, such as extreme shortness of breath or confusion. Have a plan in place for what to do in case of an emergency.

10. **Stay Positive and Encouraging:** Lastly, maintain a positive and encouraging attitude towards your loved one with emphysema. Offer praise and recognition for their efforts in managing their condition. Celebrate small victories and milestones along their journey. Your positivity and support can make a significant difference in their overall

well-being and motivation to continue managing their emphysema.

Being a caregiver for someone with emphysema requires patience, understanding, and compassion. By following these tips, you can provide the best possible care and support for your loved one while also taking care of yourself. Remember, you are not alone, and there are resources available to help you navigate this journey.

Future Research and Advances in Emphysema Treatment

As medical research continues to advance, there is ongoing exploration and development of new treatment options for emphysema. Scientists and healthcare professionals are constantly striving to improve the management and outcomes for individuals living with this chronic lung condition. In this section, we will discuss some of the exciting areas of future research and potential advances in emphysema treatment.

1. **Stem Cell Therapy:** One area of research that holds promise for the treatment of emphysema is stem cell therapy. Stem cells have the unique ability to differentiate into various cell types, including

lung cells. Researchers are investigating the use of stem cells to regenerate damaged lung tissue and potentially reverse the effects of emphysema. Early studies have shown promising results, with improvements in lung function and quality of life observed in some patients. However, more research is needed to determine the long-term safety and effectiveness of this approach.

2. **Gene Therapy:** Gene therapy is another area of research that may have implications for the treatment of emphysema. This approach involves modifying the genetic material of cells to correct or replace faulty genes. In the context of emphysema, researchers are exploring gene therapy as a means to enhance the production of a protein called alpha-1 antitrypsin (AAT), which is deficient in some individuals with emphysema. By increasing AAT levels, it is hoped that the progression of emphysema can be slowed or halted. While gene therapy is still in the early stages of development, it shows promise as a potential future treatment option.

3. **Targeted Therapies:** Advances in our understanding of the underlying mechanisms of

emphysema have led to the development of targeted therapies. These therapies aim to specifically address the molecular pathways involved in the development and progression of emphysema. For example, certain medications that target specific enzymes or proteins involved in inflammation and tissue destruction are being investigated. By targeting these specific pathways, it is hoped that these therapies can slow down the progression of emphysema and improve lung function.

4. **Lung Volume Reduction Surgery:** Lung volume reduction surgery (LVRS) is a surgical procedure that involves removing damaged portions of the lung to improve lung function and reduce symptoms. While LVRS has been performed for many years, ongoing research is focused on refining the technique and identifying the most suitable candidates for the procedure. Additionally, minimally invasive approaches, such as endoscopic lung volume reduction, are being explored as alternatives to traditional open surgery. These advancements aim to make the procedure safer and more accessible to a wider range of individuals with emphysema.

5. **Artificial Lung Technologies:** Artificial lung technologies, such as lung transplantation and extracorporeal membrane oxygenation (ECMO), are already established treatment options for individuals with severe emphysema. However, ongoing research is focused on improving the outcomes and accessibility of these interventions. For example, advancements in organ preservation techniques and immunosuppressive medications have increased the success rates of lung transplantation. Additionally, researchers are exploring the use of bioengineered lungs and other innovative approaches to address the shortage of donor organs.

6. **Personalized Medicine:** The concept of personalized medicine involves tailoring treatment plans to the specific characteristics and needs of each individual. In the context of emphysema, personalized medicine aims to identify biomarkers and genetic factors that can predict disease progression and treatment response. By understanding these individual differences, healthcare professionals can develop targeted treatment strategies that optimize outcomes for each patient. Ongoing research in this area may lead to

the development of personalized therapies and interventions for emphysema.

7. **Telemedicine and Digital Health:** The emergence of telemedicine and digital health technologies has the potential to revolutionize the management of emphysema. These technologies allow for remote monitoring of lung function, symptom tracking, and virtual consultations with healthcare providers. By enabling real-time communication and data collection, telemedicine and digital health can improve access to care, enhance self-management, and facilitate early intervention in case of exacerbations. Ongoing research is focused on optimizing these technologies and integrating them into routine clinical practice.

Conclusion

As we reach the end of this guide, I hope that you now feel equipped with the knowledge and strategies to understand and manage your emphysema. More importantly, I hope you feel empowered to take an active role in your health and future well-being.

We covered extensive information on the underlying causes of emphysema and how it impacts the lungs. You learned about the different types of emphysema and testing methods for diagnosis. We reviewed the stages of severity and the top conventional treatments, from medications to surgery to pulmonary rehab. Lifestyle changes like diet, exercise, breathing techniques, and energy conservation can make a big difference, as can complementary therapies like herbal remedies and yoga. Finding social support and maintaining motivation are crucial as well.

While it may seem overwhelming at times, take it step-by-step. Refer back to the recommendations in this book regularly to help guide your approach. Set small, achievable goals each day and week. Meet with your healthcare team consistently and keep up with all prescribed treatments. Listen to your body and notice how different therapies and activities affect your breathing and endurance. Adjust the pacing and rest periods as needed.

Above all, maintain a positive attitude and a growth mindset. Celebrate every small win, from walking five more minutes to cutting back on salt to joining a support group. Focus on all that you can do, versus what may now be limited. Let go of what you cannot control and direct your energy toward self-care. Surround yourself with loved ones who lift you up. Find new hobbies that bring you joy, even if they are adjusted for your needs. Share your experiences with others dealing with emphysema and swap advice.

While emphysema presents inevitable challenges, use every day as an opportunity to care for your body, enrich your mind, and nourish your spirit. I appreciate all that you have. Your symptoms do not define you; you are still you. Believe in your inner reserves of strength and resilience. Nobody can face emphysema alone, so never be afraid to ask for help. Listen to your healthcare providers, but remember that you are the expert on your body and needs. Advocate for yourself unapologetically.

Though emphysema cannot be cured, it can be managed, and there are always better days ahead. Take things one breath at a time, if needed. Progress may feel slow, but look back frequently, and you will see how far you've come. Draw confidence from every goal reached. Let your hopes eclipse any doubts or fears. Above all, know you have the power within to live fully and thrive in the face of emphysema.

You now have all the tools needed to move forward with purpose and possibility. I wish you the very best on your journey. Take good care of yourself and your lungs. Keep believing in better days, and they will come. You've got this!